JEAN YAXTON

WARRIOR DIET

The Ultimate Guide to Achieving the Abs of Your Dreams, Discover the Correct Diet and Effective Exercise That Could Help You Get the Body You Would Be Proud Of!

Descrierea CIP a Bibliotecii Naționale a României
JEAN YAXTON
 WARRIOR DIET. The Ultimate Guide to Achieving the Abs of Your Dreams, Discover the Correct Diet and Effective Exercise That Could Help You Get the Body You Would Be **Proud Of!** / Jean Yaxton. – Bucharest: Editura My Ebook, 2020
 ISBN

JEAN YAXTON

WARRIOR DIET

The Ultimate Guide to Achieving the Abs of Your Dreams, Discover the Correct Diet and Effective Exercise That Could Help You Get the Body You Would Be Proud Of!

My Ebook Publishing House
Bucharest, 2020

TABLE OF CONTENTS

FOREWORD

Let's face it pal. Those turtlenecks is doing anything but get rid of that double chin taking residence. On a second note, you ever feel ….

Sluggish? Out of shape? Like your clothes seem to be outgrowing you a little faster than they should? Get all the info you need here.

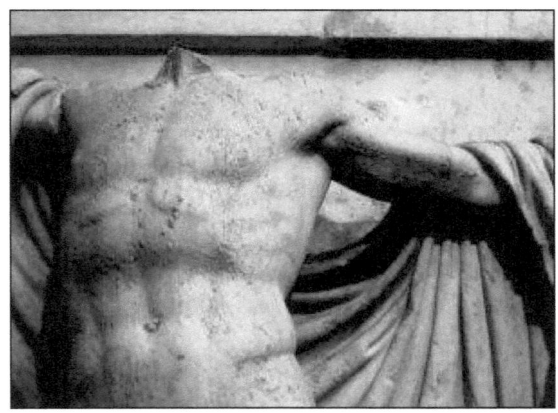

Weight Warriors
The Spartan's Guide To Chiseled Abs

CHAPTER 1

INTRODUCTION

Synopsis

Are you the guy who's perpetually perched on the couch sitting in front of the Television set eating a bowl of crisps and a bottle of beer perfectly balanced on your stomach, dreaming of that tasty, greasy Big Mac and hating yourself for it?

Are you tired of being on the heavy side? Do you want to get on the right track and for these questions to stop? Well buddy you've got it!

With this copy of Weight Warriors: The Spartan's Guide to Chiseled Abs, we'll have you out of that couch and into those running shoes in no time! Because now is the time to decide to live a healthy life-style.

The Basics

But before all else, please do keep in mind that healthy isn't being skinny. Healthy is the state of a well-fit mind, body and spirit. Not your preference on the demon scale, or how good you look in that new body hugging blouse.

It's about making the right choices that will absolutely bring amazing results throughout your lifetime. It's about giving your body the exercise and flow of positive energy it needs. It's about reinvention. Molding you into a better, happy and healthy person. The saying health is wealth was right all along.

Health is well being. Happiness that doesn't have to cost you a dime.

If you've been heavy for almost all of your life or if you have a parent who is heavy, your obesity may be highly influenced by genetic science.

But this isn't a death sentence, because I assure you exercise and a whole lot of dedication will go a long way. We can defeat the fat gene and those fat cells right here, right now.

Embracing the beautiful concept of being physically fit will come with a whole lot of great benefits, such as the amazing feeling you'll get when you wake up one morning and feel totally refreshed, better than you were before. It's like waking up on the right side of the bed every day. And once you see those pounds being knocked off on that scale, it's like Christmas came early. Now you'll finally able to get into those favorite jeans of yours that you outgrew last year or that extra mile you thought you could never make. And it gets better.

A healthy life style isn't something you can put down or pick up whenever you feel like it. It takes dedication and perseverance. In a matter of weeks, even days, you will be able to be successful and pleased with easy choices that reward you in the long run.

The toning process is extremely wonderful, giving you that extra kick and confidence everyone should have. Remember, a fit life- style is a set of selections you make day-to-day.

There is no magical formula, only dedication to making favorable selections a righteous your life. Never consider your health as something demanding or high-maintenance.

Rather, think of your health as a great investment, and not a scary project. Remember, this is you we're talking about. And don't you deserve the best life has to offer? Have self-assurance and patience and you'll be a winner by the end of this race.

List down your goals. Arrange goals for your self at steady intervals like a few weeks, to a couple of months and so forth. Be fearless. We're doing this together, step by step.

If you wish to run 5 miles within 6 months, then write it down. Don't be afraid of big dreams and high hopes. The only thing standing in the way is You. Do not expect yourself to be able to run 5 miles on the first run. You're starting off and your body isn't accustomed to the vigorous activity at hand, so don't worry.

Be easy on yourself and take it one step at a time. You won't ever get to accomplish anything if you keep telling yourself time and time again that you aren't up for it. Stop hiding from those running shoes.

Procrastination is the enemy.

Let's begin with a dietary and physical activity journal and jot down everything you consume, as well as how much physical activity you get throughout the whole day. Keeping track will help you see how much work you've done and do estimated weight changes and such.

Remember that everything adds up, from that additional café latte to taking the stairs at work. Utilize this handy journal to distinguish your sorry habits and areas for betterment.

With all the latest fitness breakthroughs and out-of-this-world diets and crazy myths, it's important to stick to the real deal. Start off with the easy bits like learning how to read nutrition labels, calculating your daily calories intake and limiting fatty food. This will help you arrive at great food selections.

Get out there and learn about chances for exercise groups and activities in your area. Walking, swimming and Yoga are awesome ways to get fit and start off your physical endeavor.

Get rid of old enticements. You are what you eat. It's time to say goodbye to the toxic food habits we don't need. The end of this relationship however has a happy ending. The procedure of living a healthy lifetime will involve breaking habits. Rather than overhauling everything you do, begin with manageable steps and get a few early wins.

Take it easy on yourself. You'll slip some of the times. You're going to crack and think about screwing this whole thing over and making a run for the closest greasy food joint in town and gorging yourself in glutton.

That's okay. Rewards are all good, and little treats from time to time are alright. Forgive yourself and indulge only when you think you've earned it.

Like a palm sized amount of Kisses that will truly satisfy you after that long run after work. But if you're constantly cheating, then you have to assess what is going on and discover ways to get back on track.

Remember that the whole story isn't on the scale. The number on the scale does not decide what kind of person you are or how pretty or ugly or nice you are either.

The scale is there to help you see the changes you need to make, and the changes you've accomplished. Weight loss might be on the top of your list, but other elements such as healthier food being consumed daily and a happier, fit you are equally just as important.

CHAPTER 2

EATING YOUR WAY TO ABS

Synopsis

When it comes to getting those flashy, A-list Abs, is your first choice to jump into that celebrity diet everyone's been raving about? Where all they take is some exotic jungle juice?

Often times a quick five to ten pounds will come off, but then pretty soon your old eating habits come right back because of the drastic changes in your eating habits.

If you're really dead set on knocking off those pounds via a diet, then you must make sure to be very devoted to it. Stick to something that you'll be comfortable with. A Diet is a life-style, not a one-time shindig.

The Food

When you're on a diet, you won't be able to eat a lot of the things that you used to. It's a sacrifice you have to be willing to make, but by the end of the day it's all worth it. But don't worry because the wonderful world of substitutes and alternatives are here to help.

In diets you might consume food you might not like a great deal and don't find comforting or easy to stomach. But that's why you need to have a diet that caters to your dietary needs.

You're going to need to be happy and comfortable with it so that you won't go quitting after a few days. Plus you'll be working out an appetite because of all the strenuous activity, so you've got to love the food.

The very word Diet already calls for a horror movie worthy scream. That's because we have this idea of diets equating to bland food and starvation, which is definitely not the case. A diet is basically just a healthier packed plate with better portions.

Therefore it's time to stop sitting in a party settling for celery sticks while all the other guests are having the time of their lives stuffing their faces with those crab puffs.

It's time to stop hiding from the social scene as food is such a big part of how we interact. When there's food presented that you'd love to eat but can't, simply because of the fear of having to sweat it out somehow while the others don't have to worry about a thing, we feel stripped, alienated, alone and insecure. It's time to stop feeling so because now, we're trying to become better. A whole new healthier and happier person.

Studies have discovered dangers in the yo-yo diet cycle of slimming down. Gaining it back plus a bit more, losing, and gaining again. It's stressful on the body to have wide sways in body weight. We think each time that we might not gain it back, but the statistics show that most of us will. And the idea as a whole is crazy and unsafe.

At the start the diet gives you a feel of control. You're taking control of your eating patterns. You might witness success as the scale drops. But soon you're fighting cravings for disallowed foods, as well as hunger twinges and a lack of energy from the lower calorie level. Finally you rise up against the diet and begin "cheating." And before long you're back to your midnight snacks and old tricks.

A relapse is something we'd all like to avoid.

Your body responds to fewer calories by decelerating your metabolism. Burning fewer calories daily is crucial in maintaining your body functions.

A slow, steady system is best to stick to. Don't rush things as your body reacts to even the slightest changes. Taking care of our bodies is of utmost importance. If you don't impart exercise along with the diet, you'll lose lean muscle mass as well as fat and water weight. When you lose muscle, your metabolic process is slowed even further and you'd have to eat even fewer calories per day to continue to slim down.

It takes a conscious effort to take a step-up with exercise when on a diet. If you don't exercise then you'll fall off of the diet, and dreadfully, the weight will come back on even quicker, as your body is burning fewer calories per day. Even worse, the weight will return as fat instead of the muscle you lost. Your body will look even less lean and healthy as it did before.

That is why every diet needs to have a harmonious relationship with exercise.

Your opening move to improve your health and appearance is to start daily exercise. The exercise doesn't have to be intense. Pick things you would like to do such as walking, biking, or swimming. Gets your body going most days of the week, leaving a day for resting up from all the toning processes your body is going through.

Find a 100-calorie change you are able to make for this week. Perhaps it's drinking one less can of cola daily, or having fat-free milk in your coffee instead of cream.

Grab a baked potato instead of that unhealthy bag of chips, or a small plate of apple and cheese instead of that butter cream cupcake. Make a 100-calorie change weekly for the next 6 weeks and you'll have made a significant alteration in your eating habits.

Don't think in terms of being deprived of the food you love, because instead you are eliminating calories you could do so much better without. By making these alterations, you are able to tip your energy balance to building and upholding lean muscle while burning and dropping off fat. Now isn't that just music to your ears?

This will be gradual instead of dramatic. You will eventually notice clothes fitting looser, your waistline shrinking, and your energy level greater. Time to go shopping for that new suite you've been dying to get into!

Friends who haven't seen you in awhile will be struck by the difference. Best of all, you didn't suffer through a grueling diet, but you fed your body right with better food options and great exercise. Way to go champ!

CHAPTER 3

THE WHY IS MORE IMPORTANT
THAN THE HOW

Synopsis

Now it's time for you to dream up fun activities instead of that super cheesy party-sized pizza. It's a little tricky, so we can start of with an easier request.

When you're thinking about what to have for breakfast, lunch or dinner, it's always good to attach some sort of physical activity that goes along with it.

For example, after dinner you can take a nice walk around the park. Drilling the idea of exercise after meals is vital for creating the perfect mindset to shed those pounds.

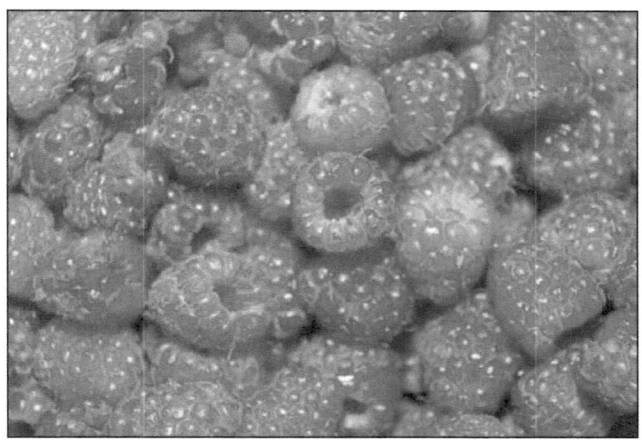

Have A Look

Change Thinking Patterns

Physical activity works best when it's a steady part of your life, and exercise at home may be much more convenient than going out of your comfort zone and attempting to find time to get to the gymnasium.

Also, physical exercise is commonly more gratifying if it takes place in a comfortable environment, and what's better than doing all the strenuous activities all in the safety and comfort of your home? Exactly.

When you start off with easy exercising patterns, you will be able to stick with it more readily and move on to more formal physical exertion more quickly.

Many of us are hooked on our automobiles, but if we simply make a little change and ditch our rides and opt to walk there ourselves, we may turn daily errands into a great work out. Instead of driving to the corner food market, why not walk or ride a bicycle?

Try exchanging your regular drive through around town with casual runs and brisk walks instead. Doing so will not only help save a lot of cash for gas but you'll also be helping Mother Nature instead of contributing to pollution. Fantastic, I know.

Take the stairs instead of the elevator in your apartment building. Walk your neighbor's dog. Join a fun run. There are so many fun ways to get fit!

If you have any kids, that's great! Kids love to move and play about. Get your kids walking around with you, and instead of packing the whole family into the mini-van, opt to walk instead. Fresh air and great exercise is wonderful.

Another great way to get as much physical activities in is through multi-tasking. Get yourself a wireless handheld and have a conversation with your friend while lifting weights. This is stealthy and effective.

Tasks that entail standing up, like vacuuming or dusting, don't need to be unappealing anymore. Plan to engage in them a couple of times each day. Utilize ankle weights and take little "walking breaks" to stretch out your legs if you are able to.

Do five or ten push-ups each time you enter or leave a room. Not too long, simply a couple of seconds to get your motor running.

A lot of people view their television set as the foe when it comes to physical activity, but it doesn't have to be that way. Think about the amount of time you spend on the sofa watching television, and then simply have yourself on a treadmill while you're watching. Presto!

Pick a particular show you love, and make it your "physical activity show," which you view while working out. Many shows are available to purchase or rent on DVD, and hour-long programs which last forty-five minutes without the commercials are the perfect length for a great workouts!

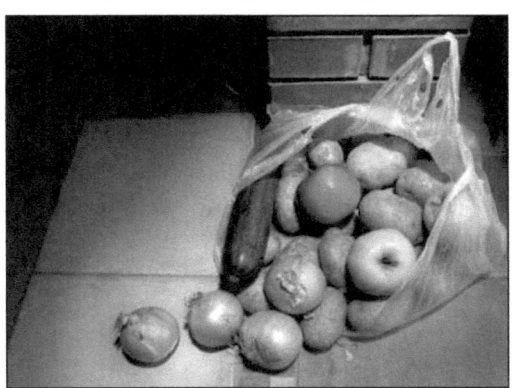

CHAPTER 4

BASIC EXERCISES FOR BEGINNERS

Synopsis

When you're out there looking for great exercise programs, you want them to be something that helps improve your over all physical appearance.

You want an exercise program that increases your total health. However, any exercise program that aims for weight reduction is neither an easy exercise nor painless route.

When the programs you take part in do not give you pain, the effectiveness of your fitness program will not at all work for shaping, toning or weight loss. When it fails, the program itself is not wrong, but the person who performs it.

No pain no gain.

Get Moving

In every exercise program, you have to know what is to be expected of you to be able to reach your goals:

1. The program must give you the motivation to sufficiently and effectively decrease the amount of calories you eat and increase the amount of calories you burn each day.

2. The program should be done in a slow, steady manner for weight loss. You have to realistically lose 1 pound weekly for the first few weeks.

3. If you have not been exercising all your life, start at a slow pace and as your body becomes adjusted, gradually increase the amount of time and the pace of exercise.

4. Choose exercises that that you enjoy and that fit your overall personality; while exercising; it is important to enjoy it at the same time.

5. The exercise program should be done regularly; as much as possible, make it as a daily routine to gain the most health benefits and weight loss. Choose those activities that fit into your schedule.

6. Exercise comfortably. Comfortable is key. If you're comfortable, you're enjoying. Enjoying the activity increases the time you choose to exercise with, burning off more fat.

7. In every exercise, your safety and comfort are your priority. Meaning, you have to wear shoes and clothes that perfectly fit in you, in such a way that you can perform well without destruction and distraction.

8. There are a lot of different exercises for you to choose from, so change daily so that you will not get bored.

9. Challenge yourself. In every exercise, it is important to increase your intensity and duration. The more you do it, the greater the effect. Also, when you have reached your goals, reward yourself to whatever your heart desires. Never lose hope of not being able to achieve your weight goal and enjoy yourself while you exercise. Make that physical activity a part of your lifestyle. Remember, if you just believe and take part in exercising, weight loss can happen, and it most definitely will.

Here are some weight loss exercise programs for you

Before starting on the exercise, do the basic warms up to prevent any cramps, torn muscles and soreness. Cool down exercises after is likewise.

Wide Squat

Stand straight and spread your legs widely. Make sure you are able to spread it with balance.

Extend your arms as in a Y position above your head.

Slowly squat down by pushing your hips back; hold into that position as long as you can and get back to the starting position.

Do 15 wide squats or as much as possible.

When you get stronger, you can be able to squat longer.

Push ups

Lie on the floor, face facing down.

Put your hands close to your shoulders.

Slowly raise your body off the ground with the help of your hands and feet as you push against the floor. Your body must be kept straight while doing this.

For beginners, you can raise your body from your knees instead of feet, reducing the work on the arms.

Do 15 repetitions; if you can't, make it 5 counts for 3 sets.

Jumping Jacks

Assume a standing position with your arms on your sides.

As you jump, spread legs and raise your arms above the head, making a circular motion as your hands meet above.

Returns to the standing position with your arms back to your sides. Do 60 repetitions or so.

CHAPTER 5

TAKING YOUR WORKOUTS TO THE NEXT LEVEL

Synopsis

This chapter steps your workouts up a notch.

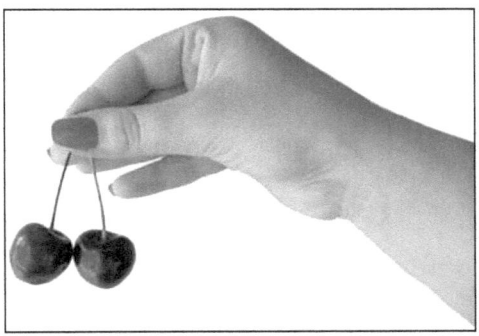

Changing It UpINTERMEDIATE

Lying Fly

- Grab two dumbbells. The weight depends on you, just not too light or too heavy.

- Lie on the floor, facing upwards.

- Slowly, raise the dumbbells to meet above your chest. Your arms must be kept straight.

- Then, lower slowly and hold just above the ground and not on the ground.

- Repeat 15 times or as long as you can tolerate.

Shoulder Press

- Almost the same with lying fly, but the difference is to hold the dumbbells at ear level.

Seated Triceps Extension

- Sit straight; hold 1 dumbbell above your head using both your hands.

- Make sure the weight is not too light or too heavy.

- Slowly lower the dumbbell behind your back, still held by both your hands.

- Keep the raised arms as vertical as possible.

- Get back to the starting position and repeat the steps for 15 seated triceps extensions.

One Armed Row

- Put your left knee on a chair, lean forward and support your body with your left arm on the chair. Hold a dumbbell in your right hand. Lift the weight by raising your elbow toward the ceiling. Hold. Return to the start. Do 15 reps.

Dumbbell Bicep Curl

- Either assumes a standing or sitting position.

- Hold a dumbbell in each hand and bring it down towards the floor.

- Slowly raise the right dumbbell toward your chest.

- Curl the dumbbell as you raise it so your palm faces your chest.

- Repeat the step, and do it on the other side. Do 15 dumbbell bicep curls.

ADVANCED

Walking Lunge with twist of torso

- Start in a standing position.

- Take a large step forward and lower your hips.

- When you are at full position, twist your upper body toward the side of the stretched leg. Twist back to the front and return to the starting position.

- Repeat steps and do it on the other side.

High Plank

- Start in a push up position, such that your hands and shoulder width apart.

- Keep your back straight as much as possible.

- Hold for 15 seconds.

Side Lunge with Arms Raised

- Assume a standing position.

- Arms should be raised straight out in front of you.

- Move your right foot to your right side and slowly lower your hips.

- Return to the starting position.

- Do 5 then repeat on the opposite leg.

CHAPTER 6

SECRET FAT BURNING TIPS

Synopsis

Some people starve themselves while others work out constantly. Some people take the expensive shortcut and have surgical interventions while others watch the hands on the clock move along as they're pounding pavement in the gym.

The truth is losing weight is hard work if you plan on keeping it off, which is inhumanly impossible. Our lives consist of eating good food, while feeling good about ourselves. Therefore we exercise to maintain the type of figure we want to have.

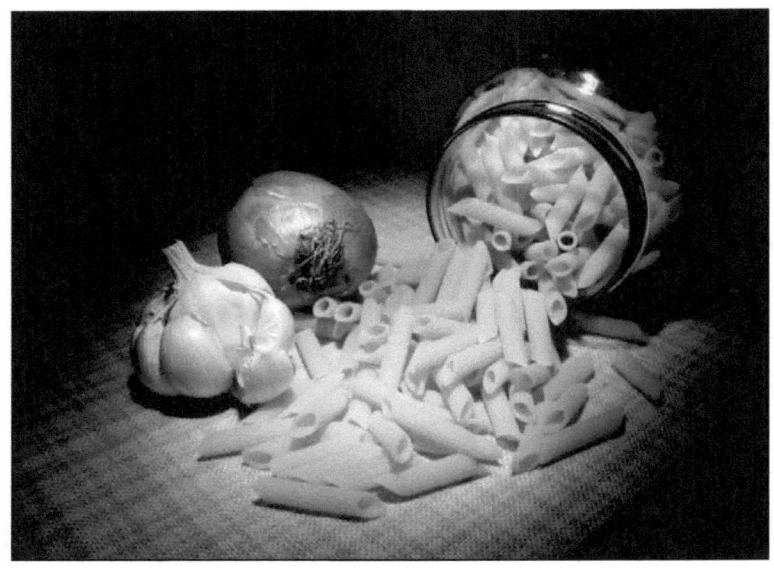

Great Info

Just because something is difficult at first doesn't mean that you won't be able to enjoy it in the long run. There's a huge difference between working hard toward something you really want, and working hard just because you feel you have to.

As stated throughout the whole book, healthy living is a choice. It is something that you are entitled to and deserve, if you're driven enough. With these super-secret fat burning tips, shedding those pounds won't seem so grueling. And when you're giving your all for the benefit of being healthy, the fruit of your labor is exquisite.

Observe:

1. Timely Eating

Eating! Everyone's favorite past time. This is the easiest thing to do, so long as you have a little self-control. Your body processes food as it consumes it, and depending on what you eat, it may or may not stop working to burn fat sooner rather than later. If you're eating a balanced diet filled with protein-rich foods and natural starches, then you're doing okay. But the frequency of eating is just as important.

Make sure you have smaller, balanced meals throughout the entire day instead of just two or three huge meals. Eating a tiny bit consistently keeps your metabolism working all day long. Little snacks through out the day also help you from eating a big serving for supper time, as it is better not to take anything passed 6 in the evening. Also observe proper eating time to limit untimely binging in the middle of the night or throughout the day. A salad after lunch can fill you up in a jiffy.

2. Make a Plan

Everyone wants to shed a few pounds and look their best. What's your goal? Losing Five pounds? Whatever your goal is, it's important to determine it early on and then form a plan for getting there. This doesn't have to be intricate. It can be as simple as saying that you want to lose one pound a week for fifteen weeks. Keeping this simple goal in mind throughout the week will help you maintain focus and clarity throughout your weight loss period. If you know the end is in sight, keep charging forward! March on, soldier!

3. Breakfast

The saying, "Breakfast is the most important meal of the day" is true! While you sleep, you're not eating, which means that your metabolism slows down considerably. When you start your day you need to start your metabolism up again and begin burning fat right away. Otherwise, your body will think it's still in a sort of hibernation mode and it will drag on and on without giving you the support you need to lose the weight. Grab a balanced breakfast every morning, filled with lots of protein and carbs so that your body gets up and running. A breakfast fit for a king if the perfect wake up call. And as the day progresses, gradually eat less. As that other saying goes, "For breakfast, eat like a king. For lunch eat like a knight. And for supper, eat like a slave."

4. Resistance

Eating right is one thing, but it won't do the job alone. You need to exercise, and one of the most important aspects of exercise is resistance training. This means hitting the gym or grabbing some weights for a good workout at home, because you should be doing this three times a week, with a day of rest in between each workout. Try to build up to 60 minute sessions and before long you'll notice a huge difference in the amount of energy you have and how much weight you're shedding.

While some of the greater mysteries in life may go unanswered for all eternity, some of the most common Earthly questions already have the answers out there. These fat burning tips are tried and true. They're proven, and they won't fail you. Just think of your goals and determine how these fat burning tips can aid you in reaching it. Can you almost see the finish line?

Wrapping Up

This way of life calls for great choices. If you're willing to stick to this course you'll discover tremendous achievements. I promise you that. This freedom provides a boundless joy that can't be attained by strains in the external world.

Delight is your natural does of goodness. It is your hallowed birthright. Everyone should be happy. We all deserve to be, and what better way than to start making these great life decisions?

Astonishing things happen when you start to align with your Self and associate your life with higher purposes in hopes of becoming a better person. You will discover so much support.

The universe has a way of affirming you and giving you what you need. Individuals and chances will start to show up everyplace. Synchronies and miracles start to occur as you begin to cut away from your toxic relationships and begin to fully give yourself to good health.

You'll know you've reached this place once feelings of serenity, harmony, and contentment are with you. Weight and food will no longer be a problem that plagues you.

You'll be gleefully engaged in the dance of life. When you're amply alive with the fierce glow of sublime contentment, you will know that you've come home to yourself.

You'll be filled wonder; the wonder that's always been inside of you, that has been waiting to shine through.

And now it most definitely can. Because now you're a whole lot healthier, confident and fit as a fiddle.

You are your own person, and you deserve better. Congratulations storm trooper! You've made it to the finish line!

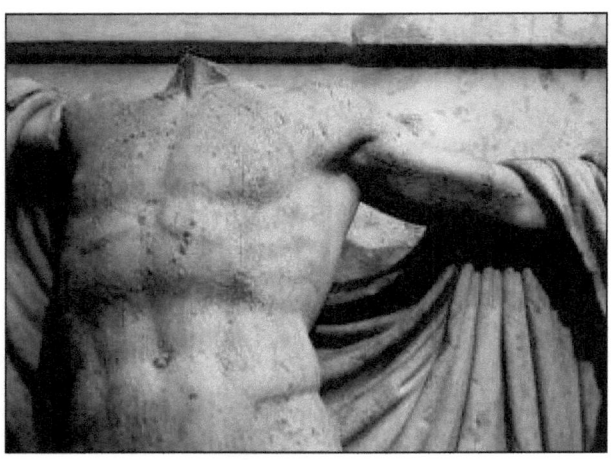

Printed by Libri Plureos GmbH in Hamburg,
Germany